VIAGRA

A Comprehensive Step By Step Guide On The Use Of Magic Blue Pill Viagra To Cure Erectile Dysfunction, Last Long In Bed In Other To Satisfy Your Partner

Dr. Cyra Brown

VIAGRA

Viagra, also known by its generic name sildenafil, is a medication used to treat erectile dysfunction (ED) in men. It was first discovered by accident in 1989 by scientists at the pharmaceutical company Pfizer, who were working on a new drug to treat hypertension. During clinical trials, they found that the drug had an unexpected side effect – it improved blood flow to the penis, leading to erections in men with ED. This accidental discovery led to the development of Viagra and its approval by the US Food and Drug Administration (FDA) in

1998. Erectile dysfunction is a condition where men are unable to get or maintain an erection sufficient for sexual intercourse. It affects millions of men worldwide and can occur as a result of various factors such as stress, anxiety, diabetes, heart disease, and low testosterone levels. Viagra works by relaxing the muscles in the walls of blood vessels and increasing blood flow to the penis, allowing for a firmer and longer-lasting erection. The active ingredient in Viagra, sildenafil, works by inhibiting an enzyme called phosphodiesterase type 5 (PDE5). This enzyme is responsible for breaking down a chemical in the body called cyclic guanosine monophosphate (cGMP), which plays a crucial role in regulating blood flow to the penis. By blocking the action of PDE5, sildenafil helps to increase the levels of cGMP, leading to improved blood flow and an erection. Viagra is available in doses of 25mg, 50mg, and 100mg, and is usually taken 30 minutes to an hour before sexual activity. It is essential to note that Viagra does not automatically cause an erection; sexual stimulation is still necessary for it to work. The effects of Viagra can last up to four hours, but this can vary from person to person. While Viagra is primarily used as a treatment for ED, it has also been found to be beneficial in treating other conditions. Some studies have shown that it may be useful in treating pulmonary hypertension, a type of high blood pressure that affects the arteries in the lungs and right side of the heart. Viagra works by relaxing the blood vessels, which can help to reduce the workload on the heart and improve symptoms of pulmonary hypertension. Another condition that Viagra may be used to treat is Raynaud's disease, a condition where the blood vessels in the fingers and toes constrict, reducing blood flow and causing them to turn white or blue. Viagra has been found to improve blood flow and decrease the frequency and severity of Raynaud's attacks. However, it is important to note that Viagra is not FDA-approved for the treatment of these conditions and should only be used under the guidance of a doctor. Viagra is generally well-tolerated, but like any medication, it can cause side effects in some people. The most common side effects include headache, flushing, indigestion, and nasal congestion.

In some cases, more severe side effects such as vision changes, hearing loss, and prolonged erections (lasting more than four hours) may occur. It is crucial to seek immediate medical attention if any of these side effects are experienced. As with any medication, there are certain precautions that need to be taken with Viagra. It should not be taken by men who are already taking nitrates for chest pain or alpha-blockers for enlarged prostate as this can lead to a dangerous drop in blood pressure. It is also not recommended for men with a history of heart problems, liver or kidney disease, or those who have had a recent stroke or heart attack. As always, it is essential to consult with a doctor before starting any new medication. Viagra has had a significant impact on the lives of men who suffer from erectile dysfunction. It has helped to improve their self-esteem, relationships, and overall quality of life. For many men, being able to achieve and maintain an erection can bring a sense of normalcy and confidence that they may have lost due to ED. Viagra has also sparked controversy and debate, with some critics arguing that it promotes recreational and casual use of the drug for non-medical reasons. Some have even dubbed it the "party drug" due to its association with increasing sexual performance. This misuse of Viagra can lead to potential risks, including increased risk of sexually transmitted infections and unplanned pregnancies. To address these concerns, some countries have imposed regulations on the sale and use of Viagra. In the US, it is only available with a prescription, and many other countries have followed suit. This helps to ensure that Viagra is only used for medical purposes and under the supervision of a doctor. In recent years, there have been advancements in the development of new and alternative treatments for erectile dysfunction, such as penile implants, vacuum pumps, and topical medications. However, Viagra still remains one of the most popular and effective treatments for ED, with over 25 million men worldwide using it.

SCEINCE BEHIND VIAGRA

The mechanism of action behind Viagra's effectiveness lies in its ability to increase the blood flow to the penis. To understand this, we must first understand the normal physiological process of an erection. An erection is a complex physiological response that involves the coordination of various systems in the body. It begins with sexual arousal, which can be stimulated by physical touch, visual or auditory stimuli, or even mental and emotional stimulation. This arousal triggers the release of a chemical called nitric oxide from nerve endings in the penis. Nitric oxide is a vasodilator, meaning it causes the blood vessels to relax and widen. In the case of an erection, this allows for the arteries in the penis to dilate and fill with blood, while the veins constrict to prevent blood from leaving the penis. This increase in blood flow to the penis creates pressure, causing it to become erect and engorged with blood. However, in men with ED, there is a problem with this process. Either there is not enough nitric oxide being released, or there is an enzyme called phosphodiesterase type 5 (PDE5) that breaks down the nitric oxide too quickly, resulting in inadequate blood flow to the penis and difficulty achieving or maintaining an erection. This is where Viagra comes in. Viagra is a PDE5 inhibitor, meaning it blocks the action of the enzyme PDE5, which allows nitric oxide to accumulate, leading to improved blood flow to the penis. It does this by binding to the active site of PDE5, preventing it from breaking down cyclic guanosine monophosphate (cGMP), which is necessary for vasodilation and relaxation of smooth muscle cells in the penis. This allows for a sustained erection during sexual activity. Viagra is taken orally and starts to work within 30 minutes to an hour after ingestion. The effects can last up to four hours, but this varies from person to person. It is important to note that

Viagra does not directly cause an erection but enhances the natural process of sexual stimulation, making it only effective when there is sexual arousal. The development of Viagra was a breakthrough in the treatment of ED, providing an alternative to invasive procedures like penile injections and implants. It has been widely studied and found to be effective in about 70% of men with ED. However, it is essential to note that Viagra is not a cure for ED, but a temporary solution. It does not address the underlying causes of ED, such as psychological issues, hormonal imbalances, or certain health conditions. There are also limitations to the use of Viagra. It is not recommended for men with certain health conditions, such as heart disease, high or low blood pressure, liver or kidney disease, or those taking nitrates for chest pain, as it can cause a dangerous drop in blood pressure. Viagra may also interact with some medications, so it is essential to inform your doctor of any other medications you are taking before starting Viagra. Aside from its use in treating ED, Viagra has also been studied for its potential use in other medical conditions. For example, it has been found to be beneficial in treating pulmonary hypertension (PH), a condition where the blood pressure in the arteries of the lungs is abnormally high. In this case, Viagra works by relaxing the smooth muscles in the blood vessels of the lungs, allowing for easier blood flow and alleviating symptoms. Another potential use of Viagra is in the treatment of altitude sickness. Altitude sickness occurs when a person ascends to high altitudes too quickly, causing a decrease in oxygen levels and resulting in symptoms like headache, dizziness, and shortness of breath.

Some studies have shown that Viagra can improve oxygen levels and alleviate symptoms of altitude sickness by increasing blood flow to the lungs.

STEPS ON HOW TO TAKE IT

Step 1: Consult with a Doctor

Before taking Viagra, it is important to consult with a doctor to determine if it is safe for you. This is especially crucial if you have any pre-existing medical conditions such as heart disease, high blood pressure, or liver/kidney problems. Also, be sure to disclose all medications you are currently taking, as Viagra may interact with certain drugs. Your doctor will be able to prescribe the appropriate dosage of Viagra for your condition and advise on any potential risks.

Step 2: Follow the Recommended Dosage Instructions

Viagra comes in three different dosages: 25mg, 50mg, and 100mg. The recommended starting dose is usually 50mg, but your doctor may adjust the dosage based on your condition. It is crucial to follow the dosage instructions provided by your doctor or pharmacist. Never take more than the prescribed dose as it can increase the risk of side effects.

Step 3: Take Viagra at the Right Time

Viagra should be taken about 30 minutes to an hour before sexual activity. It can be taken with or without food, but it may take longer to take effect if it is taken with a high-fat meal. The effects of Viagra can last for up to four hours, but it is recommended to only take one dose per day.

Step 4: Get in the Mood

Viagra does not automatically create an erection. Sexual

stimulation is still required for it to work. It is important to be in the mood and mentally prepared before taking Viagra. Relaxing and engaging in foreplay with your partner can help enhance sexual arousal and improve the effectiveness of Viagra.

Step 5: Avoid Alcohol and Grapefruit Juice

Avoid drinking alcohol before or after taking Viagra as it may decrease its effectiveness. Alcohol can also increase the risk of side effects such as headaches, dizziness, and low blood pressure. Similarly, grapefruit or grapefruit juice may interact with Viagra and increase the likelihood of side effects.

Step 6: Be Aware of Possible Side Effects

Like any medication, Viagra may have side effects. Common side effects include headaches, facial flushing, nasal congestion, and upset stomach. These side effects are usually mild and go away on their own. However, if they persist or become severe, it is important to seek medical attention. In rare cases, severe side effects such as sudden vision or hearing loss, and priapism (persistent and painful erection) may occur. If you experience any of these, seek immediate medical attention.

Step 7: Do Not Mix with Other ED Medications

Do not take Viagra with other ED medications such as Cialis or Levitra. Combining these medications may increase the risk of side effects and may lead to serious health complications.

Step 8: Store Viagra Properly

Viagra should be stored at room temperature (between 68-77 degrees Fahrenheit) and kept away from moisture and heat.

Keep it out of reach from children and pets.

RISKS AND PRECAUTIONS

The most common risk associated with taking Viagra is the development of adverse side effects. Some of the most common side effects reported by patients include headache, dizziness, flushing, indigestion, and nasal congestion. These side effects are typically mild and do not require medical attention. However, there have been cases where patients have experienced more severe side effects such as sudden vision loss, priapism (a prolonged and painful erection), and hearing loss. These serious side effects are rare but can be more prevalent in older men or those with underlying medical conditions. Another potential risk of taking Viagra is the potential for drug interactions. Viagra should not be taken with certain medications, including nitrates, as it can cause a dangerous drop in blood pressure. It is important for individuals to disclose all medications they are taking to their doctor before starting Viagra to avoid any potential drug interactions. In addition to the potential side effects and drug interactions, there are other risks associated with taking Viagra. One major concern is the use of Viagra without a prescription or without proper medical supervision. Some people may obtain Viagra illegally through online pharmacies or from friends, which increases the risk for adverse effects and drug interactions. It is crucial to obtain Viagra legally through a prescription from a healthcare provider to ensure proper dosing and monitoring. Another risk associated with taking Viagra is dependency or psychological dependence. As with any medication that improves sexual performance, there is a potential for psychological dependence on Viagra. This can lead to a reliance on the drug to achieve and maintain an erection, rather than addressing any underlying psychological or physical issues. It is important for individuals to use Viagra as directed by their healthcare provider and to address any underlying issues that may be contributing to their erectile dysfunction. There are also precautions that should be taken to minimize the risks of taking Viagra. First and foremost, it is essential to obtain a prescription from a licensed healthcare provider. This ensures that the medication is appropriate for the individual and that they are receiving the correct dosage. It also allows for proper monitoring of any potential side effects or drug interactions. It is not advisable to purchase Viagra from online sources or without a prescription as the quality and safety of these medications cannot be guaranteed. It is also important to disclose any underlying medical conditions or medications to the healthcare provider before starting Viagra. Certain medical conditions, such as heart disease, high blood pressure, or liver and kidney diseases, may increase the risk of side effects when taking Viagra. Informing the healthcare provider of these conditions allows for proper evaluation and determination of whether Viagra is safe to use. Individuals should follow the dosing instructions provided by their healthcare provider. Taking more than the recommended dose of Viagra can increase the risk of experiencing adverse side effects. It is also important to note that Viagra should not be taken more than once a day or more frequently than prescribed by a healthcare provider. Another precaution to consider when taking Viagra is to avoid the use of alcohol and grapefruit juice. These substances can interact with Viagra and increase the risk of side effects. In addition, smoking can also decrease the effectiveness of Viagra, so individuals should consider quitting smoking to maximize the benefit of the medication.

ERECTILE DYSFUNCTION

Erectile dysfunction (ED), also known as impotence, is a widespread condition that affects millions of men worldwide. The inability to achieve or maintain an erection sufficient for sexual intercourse can result in significant distress and negatively impact a man's self-esteem and relationships. Despite its prevalence, discussions about ED are often met with embarrassment and stigma, causing many men to suffer in silence. In this modern age, where the internet has made information readily accessible, it is not surprising that erectile dysfunction has become a hot topic. However, there is also a lot of misinformation and misconceptions surrounding this condition, making it difficult for men to understand and address their concerns. The first step in understanding erectile dysfunction is knowing what causes it. ED is primarily caused by problems with blood flow to the penis. Erections occur when the arteries in the penis relax and widen, allowing blood to flow in and create pressure, making the penis firm. If there is not enough blood flow or if the arteries are narrowed, an erection may not occur, or it may not be sustained long enough for sexual intercourse. Physical factors can contribute to ED, such as diabetes, high blood pressure, heart disease, and obesity. These conditions can damage the blood vessels and nerves responsible for supplying blood to the penis, leading to ED. Other risk factors include smoking, excessive alcohol consumption, and drug use. Aside from physical factors, psychological factors can also play a significant role in erectile dysfunction. Stress, anxiety, depression, and relationship problems can all lead to performance anxiety and make it difficult for a man to achieve or maintain an erection. Ironically, ED can also cause psychological issues, creating a vicious cycle of performance anxiety and further worsening the condition. While age can also be a factor in developing ED, it is not a normal part of aging. Men of all ages can experience erectile dysfunction, and it is not a reflection of their masculinity or sexual prowess. However, older men may be more likely to develop ED due to the increased prevalence of chronic health conditions and medication use. It is essential to address the topic of ED and seek medical advice as early as possible. Many men delay seeking treatment due to embarrassment or the belief that the problem will resolve on its own. However, ED is a medical condition that can have a significant impact on a man's quality of life and overall well-being. The good news is that erectile dysfunction is treatable. The most widely known and prescribed treatment for ED is oral medication, such as Viagra, Cialis, and Levitra. These medications work by increasing blood flow to the penis, helping a man to achieve and maintain an erection. They are highly effective, with success rates of 70-85%. However, oral medications may not be suitable for everyone, as they can interact with other medications and have side effects such as headache, dizziness, and flushing.

In these cases, other treatment options, such as vacuum devices, penile injections, and surgery, may be recommended. Another effective treatment for erectile dysfunction is psychological counseling. This can help address underlying psychological issues and improve a man's confidence and performance. Couples counseling may also be beneficial for addressing relationship problems that may contribute to ED. In addition to medical and psychological treatments, lifestyle changes can also go a long way in managing ED. Quitting smoking, reducing alcohol consumption, and maintaining a healthy weight can improve blood flow and overall health. Regular exercise and a healthy diet can also help reduce the risk of developing chronic health conditions that can lead to ED. While ED can be a challenging and sensitive topic to discuss, it is essential to remember that it is a common medical condition that can be successfully treated. Seeking support from a healthcare professional is the first step towards addressing the issue and improving overall sexual and mental well-being. It is also crucial for society to break the stigma surrounding erectile dysfunction.

Negative attitudes and misconceptions about ED can lead to feelings of shame and isolation for those experiencing it. Instead, we need to have open and honest conversations about this condition, providing a safe and supportive environment for men to seek help and treatment.

MEN SEXUAL HEALTH

Men's sexual health is a topic that is often overlooked and not given enough attention in comparison to women's sexual health. However, it is important to recognize that men too face various sexual health issues that can have a significant impact on their overall well-being and quality of life. In this essay, we will discuss some common sexual health problems and concerns that men may experience, as well as ways to maintain good sexual health. One of the most common sexual health problems that men face is erectile dysfunction (ED). ED is the inability to achieve or maintain an erection, making it difficult for men to engage in sexual activity. It can be caused by various factors such as stress, anxiety, relationship problems, and underlying medical conditions like diabetes, high blood pressure, or heart disease. As men age, the risk of developing ED increases, with studies showing that by the age of 40, approximately 40% of men experience some degree of ED. While ED can be a distressing and embarrassing issue, it is crucial for men to seek medical help instead of feeling ashamed or turning to unproven treatments. A doctor can properly diagnose the underlying cause and provide appropriate treatment options, such as medication or counseling. Furthermore, maintaining a healthy lifestyle by exercising regularly, managing stress, and avoiding excessive alcohol and tobacco can also improve sexual function and prevent or manage ED. Another common sexual health issue among men is premature ejaculation (PE). PE is a condition in which a man ejaculates sooner than he or his partner would like during sexual activity. It can have a significant impact on a man's confidence and cause tension in a relationship. The cause of PE is not well understood, but it is believed to be a combination of psychological and biological factors. Anxiety, depression, and relationship problems can contribute to PE, as well as certain medical conditions such as an overactive thyroid or inflammation of the prostate. Treatment for PE can include behavioral techniques such as the "squeeze" method or "stop-start" technique, as well as medication and counseling. Communication with one's partner is also crucial in managing PE and finding a solution that works for both individuals. Like ED, a healthy lifestyle can also contribute to better sexual health and potentially improve symptoms of PE. Apart from physical health, mental health also plays a significant role in men's sexual health. Men are often expected to be sexually dominant and have high levels of performance, which can lead to stress, depression, and anxiety. These mental health issues can have a direct impact on sexual function and desire. It is essential for men to address any underlying mental health concerns and seek help from a professional if needed. Another aspect of men's sexual health that is often overlooked is the importance of safe sex practices. While many believe that sexual health only refers to the ability to have an erection and engage in sexual activity, it also includes preventing sexually transmitted infections (STIs) and unwanted pregnancies.

Men should always use a condom when engaging in sexual activity to protect themselves and their partners from STIs. Regular STI screenings and communication with sexual partners about their sexual health are also essential in maintaining good sexual health. Men should also be aware of the potential risks of unprotected sex, such as contracting human papillomavirus (HPV). While HPV is commonly associated with women and cervical cancer, it can also cause health issues for men, such as genital warts and certain types of cancer, including penile, anal, and throat cancer. Men should consider getting the HPV vaccine, especially if they are sexually active and have multiple partners. Apart from physical and mental health, healthy relationships also contribute to men's sexual health. Open and honest communication with sexual partners can lead to a better understanding of each other's needs and desires, creating a more satisfying sexual experience for both individuals. Respecting and prioritizing consent is also crucial in maintaining a healthy and respectful sexual relationship.

Printed in Great Britain
by Amazon

36692461R00026